A Common-Sense View of the Mind Cure

A Common-Sense View of the Mind Cure
by Laura M. Westall

Start Publishing PD LLC
Copyright © 2024 by Start Publishing PD LLC

All rights reserved, including the right to reproduce this book or portions thereof in any form whatsoever.

Start Publishing PD is a registered trademark of Start Publishing PD LLC

Cover art: Shutterstock/Taisiya Kozorez

Cover design: Jennifer Do

10 9 8 7 6 5 4 3 2 1

ISBN 979-8-8809-0018-3

TABLE CONTENTS

Introduction 6
The Mind 7
The Brain 9
The Nervous System 20
The Emotions 25
The Imagination 29
The Attention 34
The Nature of Pain 39
The Environment 44
Conclusion 47
A Few Practical Applications 63

INTRODUCTION

Out of the night that covers me,
  Dark as the pit from pole to pole,
I thank whatever Gods may be
  For my unconquerable soul.
   It matters not how strait the gate,
  How charged with punishments the scroll,
I am the master of my fate,
  I am the captain of my soul!
            —HENLEY.

THE Western world has been slow to recognize the power of the mind over the body by reason of the fact that our philosophers from very early times regarded the mind as an independent entity—a something to be considered quite apart from the body.

"Mind can not move matter," they contended, because an impassable gulf exists between the two; and therefore a mental fact can not possibly be represented by a corresponding physical fact. The body, in their thought, was simply the chosen tenement of the soul, and operated independently of it. And this view in a modified form is maintained even to the present day by the adherents of the old psychology or metaphysical school.

But with the striking of the shackles from the insane by Dr. Pinel in France, with the work of Dr. Tuke in England and Dr. Rush in America, toward the latter half of the eighteenth century there sprang into being a new psychology, based upon the study of nerve-tissue and brain-action. The old psychology was speculative; the new is scientific. It has exchanged theory for the microscope.

By this method it was soon demonstrated that the brain is the organ of mind, and that the nervous system is the channel of communication between the mind and the external world, or the means by which man is put into relation with his environment.

The early phrenologists, in their attempts to localize brain function, popularized the former idea, while the brain-physiologists proved conclusively the indissoluble connection between the mind and the nervous system. Meanwhile the histologists, by their discovery of the nerve-cell and its p r o c e s s e s , discovered the physical basis of association of ideas and memory.

Toward the middle of the nineteenth century German scientists took up the problem; and Weber, with his law of variation, Fechner, with his psychophysical law, and Wundt, by his researches in physiological psychology, demonstrated the physical basis of mind. Henceforth psychology was to be reckoned among the natural sciences.

As was to be expected, the charge of materialism has been flung at the new by the adherents of the old school. With them, to deny the independent existence of the soul was to "rule God out of the universe." To affirm that mind and body are a unit is to negative the doctrine of immortality.

While admitting the justice of the criticism of those extremists who assert that "thought is a function of the brain" or that "the brain secretes thought as the liver secretes bile," it is unjust to that large body of monists who hold that, tho mind and body must be regarded as a unit, the soul-principle is the real ego or being, and the physical organism the vehicle of its expression or embodiment. As Dr.

Carus puts it, "Modern psychology does not destroy the soul, but merely a false view of the ego."

Accepting the position that the brain is the immediate organ of mind, and that by means of his nervous system man gets into relation with his environment, our inquiry as to the influence which mind may exert upon matter may be conducted upon both rational and scientific lines.

THE MIND

WE feel before we think; but this is merely another way of saying that mind is developed by means of sensations.

Each one of us is possest of five senses—sight, hearing, touch, taste, and smell; and if it were not for these we could acquire no knowledge. But by their operation we not only become self-conscious beings, but come into conscious relation with the world outside ourselves.

A moment's reflection will show this to be true. If, for instance, you could neither see nor hear nor touch your friend, could you form any idea of his character or personality? Would you even know that you had a friend? Or if you could neither see nor smell nor touch a rose, would not a thistle be just as acceptable?

It is unnecessary to multiply examples. The simple fact is that if it were not for the activity of the senses, each one of us would live in a world of darkness and ignorance. We would have no fuller measure of life than a jellyfish.

This is essentially the modern view. It was formerly held that each member of the human species entered upon life endowed with certain ideas—innate ideas, so-called—and hence the purpose of education, as the word implies, was to "draw out" of the mind what was already in it.

But since modern science has studied the human brain with the microscope, we have learned that this was a wrong conception, and that the mind is really a growth or development from small and poor beginnings.

The brain of the infant at birth, according to some authorities, contains all the brain cells, but they are not fully developed. No actually new cells are afterward produced. These cells by constant sense impressions are rapidly developed in the growing child.

The new-born infant can not think if he would; he is blind, deaf, and dumb—"his only language but a cry." But he can feel, and because of this, his mind begins to develop.

Thus, waves of light strike upon the retina of his eye, pass along the optic nerve to the brain, and a sight-impression is registered upon the brain; waves of sound strike upon the auditory nerve, are passed up to the brain, and in the same way a sound impression is made. And so with impressions of touch, taste, and smell.

Yet sight, hearing, etc., do not take place upon the first impact; many, many such impressions must be made before the infant consciously sees, hears, etc. For the first three months of life—what our German cousins call the dumm viertel—the brain is busy taking care of these sense-stimuli, as they are called. But just as soon as a sufficient number have been recorded, then one of nature's greatest miracles takes place: the infant looks up into his mother's face and smiles; he "crows" with delight at the sound of her voice.

Very beautiful! and quite as mysterious; for just how these sense-impressions become transmuted into consciousness we no more understand than we do chemical affinity or magnetism or gravitation. Neither science nor philosophy can solve the riddle. We merely know that all the sight-impressions are sent to one place in the brain, and those of sound to

A Common-Sense View of the Mind Cure 11

another, and smell to another, and so on; and that all these various impressions that beat upon the brain through the senses become at last elements of consciousness or mind. But this is merely the alphabet of mind-growth. Our infant must put the letters together to form words; and this is the way he does it:

When his mother holds up before him a round, bright object and says "ball," it means nothing to him—he does not understand—but if she continues to do this daily for some time, he will finally learn to "associate" the object "ball" with the word "ball," so that he will think ball when he hears the word, or sees the object. And in the same way—that is, by "association "—he learns the use to which it is put.

Now if you should put into the hands of an Eskimo an orange, and he had never before seen one, like the infant he would not know what it was or what to do with it. But your child and mine have learned by experience that an orange tastes sweet and is good to eat.

And just so, by experience—that is, knowledge gained through sensations—ideas spring up in the infant mind; and each idea associated by experience with other ideas gives rise to still others, and so on. Naturally, the broader the sense-experience the greater the stock of ideas.

It may be conjectured that the greater the stock of ideas the greater the mental confusion. But no; nature has provided for that. Just as a business man files away the letters he receives daily; just as a great manufacturer systematizes his business, dividing it into departments; just as a general organizes his army, so the mind files and systematizes and organizes its ideas; so that the adult mind has groups or clusters of ideas about art, science, politics, and so on. And what is quite to the point is the fact that these idea-clusters can get into communication with one another.

The nation is divided into cities, towns, villages, and hamlets, each distinct from the others; but a business man in Boston or New York can quickly get into communication with an associate in San Francisco or elsewhere, by mail or telegraph. And in much the same way, by what is known as "association of ideas" and memory, one idea-cluster gets into vital touch with another

Many people think that the present moment of consciousness is the mind. But this is merely a transitory phase of mind—"the stream of consciousness"—which is as evanescent as the dissolving cloud. It is necessary to mind-action and mind-growth, but the real mind is made up of the facts that we have learned by experience; and these facts are marshaled and organized into a great army of ideas, which are grouped into clusters, as we have just seen.

And this brings us face to face with a most important fact: The human mind is not a fixt, unchanging entity, but a virile, active force. How can this be proved?

One of your ideas or convictions may be that "the truth should be spoken at all times"; but I by many arguments may induce you to modify that view or "change your mind." Every day of our lives we are likely to hear some one say: "I can't believe that," or "I refuse to believe it"; yet sometimes we come to believe in spite of ourselves and thus "change our mind." And if one can thus at any time change his mind, then the ideas which constitute the mind can not be unchanging or fixt.

Now that which is permanent or fixt is in a state

A Common-Sense View of the Mind Cure 13

of rest; but that which is impermanent or changeable must be in a state of motion. Therefore the mind must be an active force, since there can be no motion without force.

Again, mind is a growth, and growth involves change, and change involves motion, and motion, force.

It is an axiom of science that "no force is ever lost," so we may well ask, what becomes of the force which we call mind?

The brain is commonly spoken of as the organ of mind; in reality, the entire body is the organ of mind, but it is upon the brain that the mind-force, or ideas in a state of activity, immediately acts. Just as the wind ruffles the surface of the water, breaking it up into waves, so the mind-force plays upon the brain and sets up waves in the sensitive tissue. In other words, the brain reacts upon the mind-force.

If you should strike your fist against the solid rock, you would feel pain. Why? Because the rock is harder than your fist and presents resistance—strikes back at you; and this striking back, as you know, is called a reaction. And so just as the water reacts upon the wind, the brain reacts upon the mind-force blowing upon it. Changes are thus made in the brain-substance. Movements of the minute particles or molecules take place, and in consequence there is a rearrangement or "reposition" of the molecules; hence it is a molecular change, and it is accompanied by a chemical change.

As a result, a new force comes into being, unlike anything else in nature. Some call it vital force, others nervous energy, or nervous fluid; but it might just as well be called mental energy, because it comes into being wholly as the result of mind or ideas acting upon the brain. And, moreover, the character or quality of those ideas tempers, colors, weakens or strengthens—in fact, varies in a hundred ways—this new energy. Indeed, it must be insisted upon that this energy exactly reflects or repeats the idea-force which gave rise to it.

But we have said "no force is ever lost," and since mind in action is seen to be transmuted into a new force by the subtle Chemistry of life, the same problem confronts us. What becomes of it?

Part of it is stored up in the brain to meet the emergencies of life; we call it reserve energy.

Another part supplies power to the muscles. A moment's reflection will show you that you must think before you act. The desire and the will to act draw from the brain the energy or power to act. Hence every movement that you make is mind in action.

The remainder of the mental energy is communicated to all parts of the body, with what effect we shall now see.

If you desire to lift a heavy weight or drive a nail, the energy to do so is provided by the joint action of the mind and brain. First there was the desire in the mind accompanied by will; and this acting on the brain caused a change in its substance and set free the energy to do just what you wanted to do. Now if you should make it your life-work to lift weights or drive nails, those muscles which you put into daily operation would develop and grow strong; that is, certain muscles and parts, being more often brought into action, would develop out of proportion to other muscles and parts, would they not? And so we come logically to another of Nature's mysteries—the law of correspondence. This being translated means that the habit of thought, desire, and will writes itself upon the physical body, because it forms the habit of life; that is, action. The mental energy communicated to certain muscles and parts gives to them a greater development. Consequently, we come finally to look and be as we think and do. There takes place what Herbert Spencer calls "a mental and physical correspondence," or "coordination of mind and body."

It is a common fact of observation. No one mistakes a clergyman for a jockey, or a college professor for a dancing-master. The avaricious man proclaims his ruling passion in his face, voice, manner, and gait; the vain or envious woman's face is set by muscular contractions plain enough to the discerning eye.

So well is this principle of correspondence understood that phrenologists, palmists, graphologists, and muscle-readers interpret the inner life and character by its aid.

But the operation of the law, as already shown, is dependent upon the reaction of the brain upon the mind-force; upon the quality and quantity of the mental energy set free by the brain; therefore, it will be worth our while to study more minutely the structure of the brain and its mode of action.

THE BRAIN

WE are accustomed to speak of the brain as the organ of mind, but it is more than that; it is the engine which runs the body—a sort of powerhouse, so to speak. The varied stock of ideas which beat upon it furnishes the fuel. If those ideas are vigorous and numerous, the engine, under normal conditions, works quickly and powerfully; but if they are weak and slow, the fire burns low—the body is sluggish.

The brain, physiologically a mass of nervous tissue, delicate and sensitive, is divided into two main parts: the cerebrum, the larger and upper, the cerebellum, the smaller, situated below and behind The cerebrum consists of an outer zone, the cortex, or gray matter, wherein lie the nerve cells forming the various centers, and an inner portion, or white substance, which consists of bundles of nerve-fibers leading from the cortical cells and distributed over the entire body. The outer surface is laid in folds or convolutions. The brain is the seat of intelligence, the organ of the conscious mind. It must act before we can take note of what is passing on.

Distributed over that portion of the cortex called the sensory area are the centers of sense-perception, which receive, respectively, the impressions of sight, sound, touch, taste, and smell. Another portion is called the motor area . Here are situated the motor centers which send out over the nerves, stimuli for producing motion. The frontal portion is known as the higher psychical area . The nerve-cells comprising these three divisions do not work independently, but are associated one with another. No cell is isolated, but each is intimately connected with some other cell, or cells, in motor and psychical area. All form part of a complex system. The stimulation of one part brings into action many other parts.

Should I touch a hot iron, the nerves of the skin receive a shock which produces a wave or current, carried along nerve-fibres to the spinal cord, thence to the brain. Pain is felt. I know I have touched a hot iron only after the stimulus has been received by the brain.

No one knows he hears a bell ring or a clock strike until the waves of sound striking the ear-drum are transmitted by the auditory nerves to the center of auditory perception. No one knows he is looking upon the face of a friend until light waves striking the retina of the eye are transmitted by the sight-nerves to the center of sight perception.

With the other parts of the brain we need not concern ourselves. As to its structure, we find that it is so sensitive and delicate that the slightest shock will cause a movement of the particles; hence all its various parts are very delicately balanced, it must be evident. They are held in equilibrium, when all is well, by nature, but it is called unstable equilibrium, because the balance is so easily disturbed. When it is permanently disturbed, we say that the person is insane; when only temporarily, we say he is irrational or hysterical.

The psychical area is so intimately connected with the various centers of the other areas, that if it becomes unbalanced, these centers, sympathizing as it were, become unbalanced. For instance, worry may affect digestion and fear may affect motion. Most of us have experienced either one or both of these conditions.

Strong emotions like anger, fear, grief, jealousy, and despair often make temporary maniacs; for they powerfully affect and disturb the equilibrium of the brain. A thing so delicate is still the engine which runs the body. One could not make the smallest movement, unless the mind supplied the force of activity. Ideas in action induce a molecular and chemical change which sets free energy not only to act but to keep the internal fires burning.

In order to heat your home you must have fuel, but you must also have a furnace or engine. If you have good fuel and a good engine, you will have a warm house. But suppose that your fuel is poor or scanty, then the fire runs low. On the other hand, suppose that your engine is worn out or poorly constructed—again you will be minus heat.

Just so, if there is a good stock of vigorous ideas there is sufficient force to insure the chemical reactions of the body—keep up the fire—but if the mind-force is weak or scanty, the fire runs low, the body is sluggish. Feeble-minded persons are slow and clumsy in their movements. On the other hand, if the brain is debilitated or worn out, again the fire runs low. So it works both ways—no fuel, no fire, or no engine, no fire.

The state of the brain, therefore, must be of equal importance with the state of the mind, as a leading English psychologist intimates when he says: "The primary essentials of health are a sound brain and a buoyant mind."

Finally, if the brain is the engine which runs the body, it must be in communication with all parts; which is true. The brain-centers govern all parts of the body; "every cell of the body has its ultimate representation in a brain-cell," which is its governor or prime mover. Thus, the cells of the stomach are represented by cells in the brain, with which they are connected by nerve-fibers; and hence your indigestion may not be caused by weakness of the stomach-cells, but by debility of the brain-cells which correspond. If the brain-cells do not work well, you can hardly expect those of the body to do so—poor engine, poor fire.

Thus we are obliged to conclude that tho we must look to the mind for the force to run the body, we must equally look to the brain as the medium for the manifestation of that force. Nature's alchemy has unvarying laws. The finest, the most vigorous mind can not work effectively through a defective medium. As well try to grow figs of thistles.

THE NERVOUS SYSTEM

WITHOUT some knowledge of the nervous system, it is impossible to understand fully how the mind may affect the body.

To begin with, as every schoolboy knows, each human being has a complex system of nerves, the fountainhead of which is the brain. From the lower part of the brain, in the back of the head, issues the spinal cord, a bundle of nerve-fibers; and from this, nerves branch out and run to all parts of the body, much as branches radiate from the trunk of a tree.

But every one does not know, or else has forgotten, that we have three kinds of nerves—those that move the muscles, called motor nerves, those which receive and carry outside impressions to the brain and called sensory nerves, and those that keep up the bodily activity, keep the fires burning—and these are called sympathetic.

Nervous centers are distributed throughout the body, some along the spinal column, others in the medulla oblongata. At certain places nerves unite forming a plexus,—the cardiac, solar, and hypo-gastric plexuses. The solar plexus is situated just back of the stomach and the hypogastric plexus in the abdomen .

"The real center of this system," says Dr. Carpenter, the English brain-physiologist, "appears to lie in the medulla oblongata [the bulb at the apex of the spinal cord], and has for its function the regulation of the blood-supply to the different parts by its action on the caliber of the arteries." That is, the great blood-channels, called arteries, which carry the red blood away from the lungs, are surrounded by a branch of these sympathetic nerves (called vasomotor), which when they contract diminish the size of the channels and hence decrease the amount of blood in them. If you should bandage your arm tightly, you would get the same result; but in the case of the nerves of which we are speaking, the action is automatic and controlled from the center at the base of the brain.

Probably the reason why these nerves were first called "sympathetic" is that if one nerve-center is shocked or does not properly conduct itself, the others sympathize, or reflex the state of the first, and then all sorts of troubles arise.

We have an analogous experience when heavy storms ravage the country. If you "call up central" on the telephone, desiring to communicate with some distant town, even tho you may "get central," you fail to reach your friend or business associate because of crossed wires, broken poles, etc.

The nervous system, like the telephone company, has its central stations from which lines radiate, and any little side line can get into touch with "central" if the intervening or allied centrals are in good running order.

So then, if there is anything wrong with the central at the base of the brain, the other centrals in the stomach or heart, for example, may become more or less unsettled and behave in a hysterical manner.

But we have said that the automatic activity of these nerves is directed from the center at the base of the brain, hence we may well ask, what directs its action?

Now we are getting down to bed-rock.

The axiom of science that "no force is ever lost"

was noted in chapter first, and here we have an illustration of it. The force, chemical and mental, which is generated by the brain through its reaction upon the mind must go somewhere. So this force follows the nerve-fibers leading from the top of the brain down to this center of which we are speaking and quickens it into action. The center automatically reacts upon the force and sends it flashing with incredible speed down the spinal cord; and thence it follows the branching nerves in every direction to the uttermost limits of the body; what is unused by the body radiates into space .

Dr. Benjamin Richardson, an English physician of the past century, claimed to have traced this radiating energy to a distance of eighteen inches from the skin; how much farther it extends we do not know.

Now, it is this vital energy spreading out over the body by means of the nerves which keeps the fires of life burning. It keeps the heart beating, the blood circulating, the stomach digesting; in fact, all the physical processes are dependent upon it. It is therefore the life-stimulus or force. And this can be easily seen. For if it ceases to flow into the arm, for instance, one not only can not move that member, but in course of time it withers. We call it paralysis.

Now if this be true, health must depend primarily upon the quality, quantity, and distribution of this vital energy; for if it depreciate in any respect, all the physical processes are weakened. And if there be a weak spot, there it will be felt to the greatest extent. And there generally is a weak spot. Few, if any of us, are built like the "Wonderful One-Hoss Shay"!

But there is still another phase of the matter.

We have seen that the nerve-center in the

A Common-Sense View of the Mind Cure 23

medulla regulates the supply of blood in the blood-channels and also in the blood-vessels of every organ or part. And this it does automatically according to the needs of the various parts. Thus, in good health, the thought or smell of food and the act of eating quicken the nerves of the stomach and cause the blood-vessels to expand and fill with blood. And then the digestive secretions pour into the stomach, ready to digest the food. On the other hand, the thought of danger so shocks the automatic center of the brain that the heart, with which it is connected by large nerves, may be temporarily paralyzed.

Hence it must be clear that all the functions of the body are dependent upon the activity of these nerves, which increase or cut off the blood-supply according as the brain is affected. If there is nervous exhaustion, the circulation is weak; consequently there ensue "functional disorders."

Also it follows that if the supply of blood to any organ or part is depleted, the nutrition of that part will be impaired. For the blood-stream contains the elements of nutrition by means of which the tissues are constantly built up. The daily tissue-waste can be repaired only through the blood, and hence the ultimate integrity of all parts depends upon the supply of blood, and also the quality of the blood. For if the blood contains impurities, the parts can not be renewed any more than you can repair a garment with rotten cloth or build a house of decayed wood.

To sum up: From this sympathetic nerve-center at the base of the brain, the mental or life-energy liberated by the brain passes by way of the spinal cord and nerves to all parts of the body, giving life or quickening into action each and every part. It controls the supply of blood to all parts, varying it at need. Without it all physical processes would cease; and upon its presence depends the circulation of each part and consequently the healthy condition of each part.

And thus become apparent two fundamental essentials of health: the quality, quantity, and distribution of the vital energy and the blood.

It is now plain what becomes of the force generated by ideas in a state of action. First, they play upon the brain, as the wind plays upon the water; this sets up waves or currents in the brain-stuff; the molecules are displaced or rearranged, and this sets free a new kind of force, which must be mental, since the mind begot it.

This mental energy then flows down from the brain; like the sap rising in the tree and penetrating to the outermost twigs, it flows by way of the nervous system to the extreme limits of the body. And it is the life-force, since, if it is impaired, all the vital processes are weakened.

THE EMOTIONS

IT must be clear from what has already been said that in order to conserve health it is necessary to maintain unimpaired the mental energy, or, as it is sometimes called, the vitality. It will be well, therefore, before proceeding further, to inquire as to what agencies tend to impair it.

The answer is, broadly speaking, anything which fatigues or depresses or profoundly shocks the mind.

You know how fatigue "takes the life out" of one. The reason is not far to seek. Whatever we do, we do first mentally; unless one "puts his mind on his work" he can not do that work successfully. And this mental effort stimulates the brain, keeps it pumping energy to the muscles, until finally the muscles refuse to act, because both mind and brain are fatigued. And this fatigue, it is said, generates a poison which affects the blood.

To continue to whip up the muscles by pure force of will when this point is reached is sheer folly. Yet we see it done every day, and regardless of the knowledge that under such conditions the system is an easy prey to disease.

Lack of sleep also greatly depletes the vital force, but this is so well known as hardly to need mention. Anxiety or worry has the same effect. Some authorities say it breaks down the brain-cells, and in many cases through its effect on the solar plexus it acts either as an emetic or a cathartic.

Equally devitalizing are certain emotions. Take anger, for instance. At first, there is a marked increase of energy, owing to the fact that the emotion appears to charge the brain electrically—the reserves are called out! This sets free a tremendous current of vital force, which swoops down upon the sympathetic nerve-center, affects the heart, and deranges the circulation, and through its action on the solar plexus interferes with digestion. As the emotion subsides, this force, otherwise unexpended, radiates into space and then ensues exhaustion. It is a sort of cyclone, which not only deranges the physical processes and takes the strength but acidulates the blood.

Then there is fear, which, as everybody knows, sometimes causes death. Sudden and violent fear powerfully affects the heart, causing exhaustion and occasionally instant death. Its effect upon the blood is also apparent, for it has been known to turn the hair white in a single night.

Prolonged grief and despondency by depressing the mind weaken the brain and retard the circulation; thus by degrees the vitality is sapped. "Dying of a broken heart" is no chimera of the imagination.

"Each strong emotion," says Herbert Spencer, "affects the activity of the heart, and with it we have the accompanying gush of nervous fluid, spreading along the vasomotor nerves, which changes the state of the arteries throughout the body. . . . It also disturbs the intellectual balance—nervous fluid is drafted off."

It does not seem to be generally understood that strong emotions unbalance the mind, and of course the brain; but a little reflection shows that this is true. An angry person will not "listen to reason," because his reason is overwhelmed by emotion. In other words, he is "beside himself"—hence we speak of "insane rage."

The same is true of fear. Let a man's life be jeopardized, and he may at once lose all consciousness of moral obligations. The panics which occur on steamboats and in fires are illustrations.

Extreme jealousy is a kind of madness.

Shakespeare in "The Winter's Tale" shows how impossible it is to convince a jealous person that his suspicions are unfounded. The poor victim has lost his mental perspective—he "can't see straight."

In view of these facts, it is obvious that in order to preserve the vitality—that is, hold stored up in the brain a reserve of mental energy—one must acquire and practise self-control. It is not always possible to avoid sudden grief or fear, but the habit of self-control, once established, gives one the power to minimize all catastrophes. It is always possible by the practise of self-control to vanquish anger, jealousy, and despondency. Many persons are emotional spendthrifts; they fritter away their life-energy by giving full rein to their emotional nature, and as a consequence have nothing left with which to meet the emergencies of life. Their account in the bank of nature is overdrawn. Is it any wonder that they succumb readily to disease?

But self-control does not necessarily imply the stifling of all emotion; let us be human beings, not clams. An existence which knows not all the deepest emotions that the human soul is capable of feeling and expressing is only a poor travesty of life. The point is to control, rather than be controlled by, one's emotions.

However, to our satisfaction and for our salvation there is a class of emotions which is in sharp contrast to those discust, because distinctly vitalizing. There is cheerfulness, for instance, and contentment. All our psychologists, physiologists, and physicians are agreed that cheerfulness, contentment, hope, joy, and happiness are the best tonics in the world, the true balm of Gilead or elixir of life. It is not surprizing, therefore, that the society of the cheerful person is eagerly sought.

THE IMAGINATION

WE think in pictures.

Each idea which is presented to the mind forms a picture. Thus, if I say, "I hear a robin singing," a picture of a redbreast on the branch of a tree, with his throat swelling with song, will probably form in your mind. Or if I should say, "The sea is blue to-day," a vision of a wide expanse of blue water, with white-capped waves shimmering in the sunshine, will appear to you.

Why is this?

We saw in chapter first that it was not so in the beginning; our ability to form mental pictures is due to what is called "association "—object with sound, sound with object, etc.—and that the wider our sense-experience, especially in early childhood, the greater our ability to form concepts or pictures. We thus get a glimpse of how imagination may be cultivated.

How important it is in life we can in part realize by reflecting how essential it is to art, music, literature, science, invention, and discovery.

Thus: The artist sees mentally his picture or statue as it is to appear before he has touched brush or chisel.

The architect sees the cathedral fully completed "in his mind's eye" before the ground is broken for the foundation.

The musician hears the cadences of his symphony before he has written a line of the score, and did not Columbus have imagination? And Watts, Bell,

Darwin, and Marconi?

In fact, starting with the savage who naturally and appropriately exprest his thoughts in "picture-writing," the civilization of to-day has become what it is largely through the imaginative power of the human mind.

The relation which imagination sustains to the mind is so intimate as hardly to permit of dissociation. It would seem absurd to say imagination is mind, yet if we think in pictures, if the component elements of ideas are pictures, which is imagination and which is mind or thought? Take our concept of God, for instance. Where is the person who can think of God as a pure abstraction? If we take away the form in which imagination clothes our concept, what is left?

This may seem a digression; but in reality it serves to show how impossible it is for us to think except in pictures.

That is why, when we think of ourselves, we form a picture in our minds of ourselves. It differs from the picture others form. No one has the gift to "see himself as others see him," but true or false it is vitally important. Since every idea must clothe itself in some form, then the influence of ideas upon the mind—that is, the reasoning faculties—must be largely determined by the form in which they present themselves.

For instance: You are walking through the woods and inadvertently step upon a crooked stick which curls up around your ankle. Instantly you think "snake," for a picture of a snake twining around your ankle forms in your mind.

Now, one of two things will happen: If you are in the habit of controlling yourself, acting upon reason rather than impulse, you will stop and investigate.

A Common-Sense View of the Mind Cure 31

If not, your imagination will swamp your reason, and you will believe "snake," scream, and run.

Or again: Suppose that you array yourself in your finest raiment with a view to attending some social function at which you wish to look your best. Before leaving home, you survey yourself in the mirror with satisfaction, deciding that your appointments are in perfect taste and harmony, even elegance, and go forth to bewilder all beholders. But arriving on the scene, you meet an acquaintance, who, after looking you over with a critical eye, turns away with an expression which plainly says: "Poor thing! Why doesn't she learn how to dress?"

Immediately you shrink in your own estimation. The mental picture which you have formed of yourself changes color and shape. You no longer see yourself as well-drest, but as shabbily and inartistically arrayed.

Now, suppose that a man forms a mental ideal of himself as fortunate, successful, popular, happy, and well. The mental state which results colors the mental energy and this spreading out over the body creates chemical changes. And thus we have the phenomenon of correspondence. We see it in the expression of the face, voice, manner, and bearing. He walks with an elastic step. He greets his acquaintances buoyantly. He is at peace with himself and all the world.

But let one form the opposite ideal. Let him picture himself as unfortunate, unsuccessful, unpopular; unhappy, and ill. Do you doubt that a corresponding effect will be produced? Will not his countenance be downcast, his manner shrinking, his step heavy and slow? Will he not appear to feel that he has one foot in the grave?

The simple fact is that to imagination is due most

of our suffering. As Hubbard says: "We suffer in proportion as we have imagination."

A little child or an animal recovers very quickly from an injury or illness simply because they lack the imaginative power to conjure up a vision of pain or death. When actual pain ceases, they cease to think about it and to fear or fancy its return.

And this explains why through imagination one may make himself ill or cause his own death. Temperament usually, tho not always, enters into the case. Those persons who have what is called the hysterical temperament have an ill-balanced mind and brain. The emotional nature is apt to be stronger than the intellectual, and so upon very small provocation imagination may submerge reason. Hence a slight pain or uneasiness may be mentally magnified into a mortal disease. Naturally, their sufferings are intense, but they themselves are unwittingly responsible, since they make no effort to control the morbid reaction of the mind.

It is evident, therefore, that uncontrolled imagination unbalances the mind; the images which it presents are distorted; they are not true images. The reasoning faculties are the balance-wheel of the mind. When we are perfectly sane, we submit each idea to the test of reason; but when emotion or imagination colored by fear has us in its grip we can no longer reason.

For instance: You are passing a lonely graveyard alone, at the mystic hour of midnight. You may not have thought of ghosts at all; indeed, you may regard such a belief as a vulgar superstition. Nevertheless, when a figure clothed in white rises up from among the graves, or appears to do so, and glides toward you, it is ninety-nine chances out of a hundred that you will take to your heels and not

A Common-Sense View of the Mind Cure

trust yourself to look behind.

On the morrow you will be disgusted with yourself. You will recognize that the uncanny sensation caused by association of ideas—graveyards, death, and wandering shades—set your imagination at work and prevented calm judgment from acting. In other words, your mind was unbalanced by the picture which fear caused fancy to paint. We see this often where highly imaginative children are frightened by some person or thing; it seems almost impossible to convince them that the object is not what they think it is.

Well, "it is a poor rule that won't work both ways." If the power of imagination is so great that it may cause disease, then by that same token it should cure disease. As a matter of fact, no one can faithfully test it without becoming convinced of its usefulness. Since, as we have seen, the body tends constantly to echo the mental picture one entertains of himself, then if one is not well, it is essential that he should overhaul his mental picture-gallery; cast the old "as rubbish to the void," and hang up new ones, fresh from fancy's brush, imagining himself as he wishes to be—fortunate, happy, and well.

THE ATTENTION

YOU are walking through the city street, thinking of nothing in particular, watching the passing throng, glancing idly about. But suddenly you stop short with your gaze riveted upon a shop window—something therein has caught your attention.

Most of the time our minds drift. Tho there is a procession of images or ideas passing constantly across the field of consciousness, we give no heed to any one of them, but, like a leaf on the stream, float idly along. However, we have the power to single out one of these ideas and fix the whole mind upon it. And this is attention; it is holding one idea in consciousness to the exclusion of other ideas.

Now, thus to fix the mind wholly or concentrate attention upon a single object of consciousness is to get a clearer idea of it. We see it in all its details, a more distinct mental image of it appears to "the mind's eye," and it takes a stronger hold upon the mind.

For instance: A friend has made a remark which has hurt your feelings. If you fix your mind upon it—that is, think about it constantly—it gains a stronger hold upon your mind and you suffer correspondingly. Or, if you have a hole in your glove and fix your mind on it—keep thinking of it and looking at it—it will look bigger and bigger to you, until you think everybody you pass in the street is noticing it.

And the . same is true of sensations. Suppose you

A Common-Sense View of the Mind Cure 35

have a pain. If you attend to it, think about it, and talk about it, it will grow worse, until after a while you will not be able to think or talk of anything else. As a matter of fact, the minds of many persons become unbalanced by much thinking and talking about their ills. We call it hypochondria.

This brings us to a very curious and, to many, incredible fact. If one fixes his attention upon some part of his body, he will in a short time perceive uneasy sensations arising therein; if he continues to do so, he may produce first pain and finally disease.

It has long been known that if the morbid attention becomes fixt upon some part of the body, actual disease may be induced. The celebrated Dr. Tuke, of England, said more than a century ago that "if the attention be directed toward any bodily organ, abnormal sensations may be perceived in it and disease may be developed."

We do not have to go far afield for the explanation; fear and imagination color the mental energy which the act of attention sends flying to the spot. Thus: You think of your foot, and as the electric power-house sends the current along the wires into your house, so the brain sends the mental current through the nerves to your foot. Ten minutes more or less will suffice to incite sensations. If there is pain in the foot, it will be augmented: or if you imagine pain, you can excite pain. For the current is colored or tinged by your state of mind; and if fearful imagination control your mind, you may, by persistent direction of attention, induce disease in your foot.

Says Dr. James Braid: "A strong direction of consciousness to any part of the body, especially if attended with the expectation or belief of something about to happen, is sufficient to change the physical action of the part. Thus, every variety of feeling from an internal or mental cause, such as heat or cold, pricking, creeping, tingling, spasmodic contractions of the muscles, catalepsy, attraction or repulsion, sights of every form or hue, colors, tastes, smells, etc., may be excited. Moreover, the oftener such impressions have been excited the more readily may they be reproduced by the laws of habit and association."

Quotations from many eminent men might be adduced to enforce this point, but one from Dr. Carpenter must suffice: "The volitional direction of consciousness to a part suffices to call forth sensations in it, which seem to depend upon a change in its circulation; and if this state is kept automatically by the attraction of the attention, the change may become a source of modification not only in the functional action, but in the nutrition of the part." And if such a change is expected, as Dr. Braid suggests—that is, if the "expectant attention" is aroused—the result is much more marked.

So if one is suffering from indigestion, and thinks he has eaten something indigestible, he unconsciously directs his attention to his stomach, and watches for, or expects, the symptoms. From what has just been said, it is easy to see why he is unlikely to be disappointed!

Well, as with imagination, "it is a poor rule that won't work both ways." If morbid attention and imagination can cause disease, then a sane, intelligent use of them should cure disease.

Let us see how it works out.

In the chapter on the nervous system it was said that if the mental energy or vital force was depleted or unequally distributed the weakest spot would be the first to suffer.

A Common-Sense View of the Mind Cure 37

Now, suppose that your stomach is your weak spot. The nerves in the walls of your stomach (vasomotor) are unable to perform their functions because of an insufficient supply of force, consequently the circulation "lags superfluous"; there is not enough blood in the blood-vessels for the glands to secrete the gastric juice. Very well, then. By fixing your attention upon your stomach, you send to the nerves an increased supply of vital energy; this will set them at work; the blood-vessels will then fill with blood, and the blood will bring to the cells sufficient nutrient materials to cause the secretion of the gastric juice. Your stomach will then begin to disgest the food, and if this be kept up for twenty minutes, let us say, the sensation of fulness, weight, cold, and the gas, caused by fermentation, will all pass off. If in addition to attention you "suggest" that your stomach is strong or imagine that it is, the result will be more satisfactory.

This is no idle dream or vagary of fancy. It is based upon well-known laws of physiology and psychology, and repeated experiments have demonstrated its practicability. That such a use of attention changes the physical action of the part involved we have scientific confirmation. Professor Gates, of the Smithsonian Institution, says, in effect, that since the brain-centers govern all parts of the body and are in direct or indirect control by means of fibers with every cell of the body, one can by practise learn to send a strong stimulus to any cell or collection of cells. This stimulus is vital force or mental energy, and when it reaches its goal, it causes a physical change; for it "alters the chemistry of the secretions and excretions, and the thermic and lymphatic functions."

In other words, this action causes a change in

nutrition, for if we increase the supply of blood to any part, we offer it more nutrient material with which to improve flagging function and rebuild wasted tissues.

This makes it easy to see why, when the morbid attention is fixt upon some organ, it is possible to develop disease in it. Fear and imagination, as has been said, so color the vital force as to paralyze the nerves and that stops the circulation, which of course interferes with nutrition.

The effect of an act of attention, it is evident, depends upon the mental state. If the mind is morbid—that is, charged with fear, anxiety, and disordered imagination—the effect is vicious; but if the mind is sane—that is, under the control of reason—the effect is salutary, particularly if the act of attention is charged with the belief that good is going to result. And that result may be augmented and expedited by painting a mental picture of the desired result.

THE NATURE OF PAIN

THERE is a great deal going on around us of which we are wholly unconscious, for the reason that nature has set limits to our perceptive powers. There are sounds which we never hear, sights which we never see, things which we can not touch, etc.

The explanation usually given is that all the forces of nature, such as light, heat, sound, and electricity, have a vibratory motion, but our brains are able to react only upon a limited number of such vibrations—those within a certain range. When they exceed that limit—that is, greatly increase or diminish the vibratory rate—we either do not perceive them at all or else they occasion us physical discomfort. Thus, a low sound has a slow rate of vibration; we do not hear it distinctly; a shrill sound has a high rate of vibration, and if near at hand is unpleasant or hard to endure.

A block of marble is cold, but one can hold his hand upon it comfortably; a block of ice is very cold and if one attempts to hold his hand upon it, he experiences an unpleasant sensation. The sound of a violin is agreeable, but the sound of a steamboat whistle gives a sensation of pain.

So then those vibrations which are within a certain range we find pleasant, but those that exceed that range we find painful.

Pain, then, must be an unpleasant sensation, and sensations are always mental. Hence pain must be mental.

Now, in chapter first it was noted that a stimulus

or sense-impression made on the brain first resolved itself into sensation—we feel before we think. Thus, I touch a hot iron. The impression made upon the nerves in my finger-tips must travel up the arm to the brain, where another impression is made. That impression gives rise to a feeling or sensation in consciousness, and then the mind says: "That iron is hot. I have burned my finger. Oh, how it hurts!"

A strong impression was made on the delicate nerve-tissue of the brain, too strong to be agreeable, and the mind calls it pain. But not until consciousness perceived the stimulus did I feel the pain or know that I had burned my hand.

So, you see, not only is pain a sensation, but it must be mentally perceived before we know that it is pain. In other words, pain is mentally perceived sensation. It matters not whether the sensations originate externally or internally, the fact remains.

An illustration or two will make this clear.

Suppose you are suffering with neuralgia, but having tickets to the theater and being eager to hear some noted actor, you resolve to go. Now, when you take your seat you will perhaps think that you will not be able to sit through the performance. But the curtain rises. The beauty of the stage-setting and the movement of the drama absorb your attention, and not until the curtain falls do you feel any pain. Why? Because your mind has been so absorbed by what was passing on the stage that you did not think about your pain and hence did not perceive it.

Again: You are prostrated by a headache. Somebody below stairs or in the next house cries "Fire!" and instantly you are on your feet, your whole mind absorbed in locating the fire and aiding to extinguish it. And not once, till the excitement subsides, do you remember your pain. Where was it

A Common-Sense View of the Mind Cure 41

when you were not thinking of it?

Obviously we have to think pain before we know that it is pain, and so we are obliged to conclude that pain is not in the nerves or organs or tissues of the body, but in the perceiving mind—that is, it is mental—a recognized or perceived sensation.

You may say, "Don't you suppose I know when I have a pain in my foot?" Yet the pain is not in the foot; it is a perceived sensation which imagination refers to the foot.

How can that be? Thus: The nerves in your foot for some reason or other are irritated; they protest and that starts a vital current up the nerves of the leg to the brain and there a corresponding irritation is set up. The mind perceives the irritation and then imagination steps in and refers it to the source of the irritation. The cells in the brain which correspond with the foot are in telegraphic communication with one another, and thus it is very natural to infer that the pain is where the primary irritation is; whereas we perceive the irritation and call it pain. If one has not thought about this matter, it may seem improbable, but there are not wanting facts to substantiate it.

For instance, if you should sever the nerve-trunk in the leg and thus interrupt communication with the brain, your foot might be pinched or pricked or burned and you would feel no pain. Or if you should cut the nerve between the little finger and the brain, the surgeon might amputate your little finger and yet you would feel no pain.

Or your arm might be rendered cataleptic by "suggestion," and you would not then feel a pin which was passed through the skin.

On the other hand, if the cells in the brain which correspond with the foot were irritated in some way, you would think you had a pain in the foot. Even if the foot were amputated, you would think you had a pain in the imaginary foot or where it used to be. Again, you may have a pain in one knee, or think you have, and develop a sympathetic pain in the other knee. But if the pain is in the knee, why the sympathetic pain? Simply because the brain area which corresponds with and governs both knees is irritated, and imagination does the rest.

So there is really no escape; pain is mental, or a perceived sensation.

Well, if pain is mental, the more one thinks about it the more he suffers, which every one knows is true. To fix the attention upon it, as we have seen, is to give it a stronger hold upon the mind. Therefore, if one diverts his mind from himself, he diminishes his sufferings.

Some say, ignore pain. This is excellent advice if one can follow it. "There's the rub." The difficulty is that the immediate effect of severe pain is temporarily to unbalance first the brain, then the mind. It acts very much like a strong emotion. The brain-cells seem to be paralyzed, the reasoning powers, self-control, and will are temporarily submerged, and thus the door is open for emotion. And it comes, cavorting to the front like a war-horse. See how quickly fear and imagination begin to work! Note how unreasonable and irritable and weak-willed the average person is under the influence of pain. Therefore, one must have a well-disciplined mind and strong will to be able to ignore severe pain.

Yet it is moral cowardice to be always whimpering when one is hurt. And the more one yields to pain, the more it enslaves him; the more difficult it is for him to "rise above it." How, then,

A Common-Sense View of the Mind Cure 43

shall we crack this nut?

Undoubtedly, it is necessary to cultivate moral heroism. If we teach ourselves to make light of trivial discomforts, we may, by degrees, so discipline our minds as to be able to master great ones. If one persistently fights back at it, he will by degrees lessen the receptivity of the upper brain (cortex) and thus throw the stimulus back upon the lower part of the brain, of whose operations we are unconscious. By persistently refusing to admit it, one may prevent it from gaining so great a power over his mind; it rebounds from the seat of consciousness as a ball rebounds from an unyielding wall. Thus, in time, a measurable degree of control will be acquired over the seat of consciousness; it does not respond so quickly to that particular stimulus.

Needless to say it can not be done in a day, but it is a moral victory, a phase of self-mastery well worth working for, and above the price of rubies.

THE ENVIRONMENT

LIFE is series of reactions upon environment. In other words, the self-existent principle of life perpetuates itself by reacting upon natural forces which play upon it.

Just as the life-principle in the plant reacts upon the chemical elements of the soil, the air, sunshine, heat, and moisture, so the life-principle in man reacts upon and thus assimilates food, drink, air, light, heat, etc., which are elements of his environment. And man is as dependent upon these natural elements as is every other living being. To ignore it, to deny the part it plays in his existence, is to cut the ground from under his feet.

For man is not an isolated fact of nature. "He is as much a part of the cosmos," says Huxley, "as the humblest weed"; and like the seed sown upon stony ground which can not spring up and put forth, he can not attain his best development amid unfavorable conditions.

Experience has taught him that certain elements are necessary to sustain life: pure air, pure water, pure food, sunshine; and given these constituents in proper proportion, there exists a sound basis for health, as the automatic activity of the brain and nervous system controls assimilation and nutrition.

But if through negligence, ignorance, poverty, or a wrong habit of life, one or more of these elements are lacking or inferior in quality there result impoverished blood and enfeebled vitality.

Now the common sense of every person should

tell him that no mental power can reinstate health if the environment is unfavorable or the laws of hygiene are constantly violated. Man is finite, not infinite; hence the human mind can work no miracles. It works successfully only in harmony with nature's laws; but the operation of those laws may be assisted by intelligent adaptation to the environment.

This gives free play to that healing force of nature—called by medical men vis medicatrix naturæ—implanted in every living thing. Thus the bruised plant, the sick or wounded animal, through its agency, regain their normal state; the surgeon sets the broken bone, but nature reunites the severed parts.

And this is a cosmic force, ever struggling to reinstate health and preserve life; and in many cases it will do so, without other aid, if the sufferer will assist nature by the exercise of intelligence and self-control.

It must not be forgotten, however, that there is a mental as well as a physical reaction upon external forces. Man is a two-sided phenomenon, on the one side mental, on the other physical. Both are important factors in the equation; both are essential to his existence as a human being.

But while no amount of thinking will change impure air into wholesome air, or avert its pernicious effect, or render adulterated food nutritious, yet there are cases where the mental reaction is so poor that even the best conditions fail to conserve health.

Take the "grouchy" man, for instance, who complains that his food is not well cooked or else indigestible; who grumbles at the weather, at the streets, at the transportation companies, at his neighbors, his family, etc. Such a man would be neither well nor happy in the Garden of Eden, for his mental reaction upon life is morbid and the effect of this upon all physical processes vicious.

The fact is one may get such into a "state of mind" as to pervert all of nature's processes and nullify not only the spontaneous effort of nature to preserve life and health but every hygienic and medical agency which can be employed.

And so, when all is said, we must conclude that the mental reaction is as important as the physical. Life is a double reaction upon nature—or a two-sided phenomenon; both sides are necessary to the perfect whole.

But the real essentials of life on the physical side are few: air, water, sunshine and food, shelter and clothing. Of these, the first three are, generally speaking, the gifts of nature; and assuming that they are within reach, then one may by intelligent effort so mold and adapt himself to conditions, or so improve conditions, as to attain both health and happiness. Some of the world's greatest leaders flowered from poverty and squalor.

CONCLUSION

IT is impossible to state at this moment just what the limitations of mind-cure are. It has been little more than half a century since the subject was lifted out of the realm of the occult and placed upon a scientific basis, tho for most persons it still possesses a mystic character. Much has been learned, but there is undoubtedly much more to learn; we are still merely "nibbling around the edges."

Less than fifty years ago there were few physicians who believed that disease could be cured by mental influence; to-day there are clinics in many European cities, and leading physicians of America are using it in one form or another.

At present the medical fraternity takes the ground that only mental, nervous, and functional disorders are amenable to mind-cure. Its future, therefore, seems to hinge upon the distinction between functional disorders and organic affections. On this point Dr. Schofield, of London, says in his "Force of Mind" that the more we examine this distinction, the more it tends to disappear; while another authority says: "There is no disease which does not involve organic change somewhere "—which seems reasonable. For we know that no organ can perform its functions if the nervous action is weak, and the lessened blood-supply impairs nutrition. Would not cellular degeneration finally ensue?

If this process could be arrested in its incipient stage, and functional action and nutrition improved by a combined medical and mental treatment, or by the latter alone in the manner already indicated, the probability is that the parts could be built up.

Dr. Gayer, of New York City, at the head of a new movement looking toward further investigation, claims that under hypnosis several cases of organic affection have been cured recently—if we are to trust the press—and also a severely burned arm healed.

The latter does not seem surprizing when we remember that under hypnosis French physicians have raised blisters on various parts of the body, have caused drops of blood to exude from the skin and even the name to appear, written in letters. of blood upon the arm.

Dr. Carpenter, in "Mental Physiology," describes a cure of warts by simple "suggestion," and the daily papers report that there is living to-day in a Boston suburb a man who cures such excrescences by simply passing his hand over them. Corns have also been cured by suggestion.

As regards structural changes, it is an open question. The distinguished Frenchman Camille Flammarion asserts that the entire body may be caused to undergo change within a year; the softer portions yielding in from one to three months, the harder portions requiring eleven months.

In apparent confirmation of this we have Mailer's law: "A structural defect tends to be removed by an act increasing the organic action of the part."

And that this may be a mental act, Dr. Laycock points out, for he says: "If the attention be daily directed to an opaque cornea during a hypnotic trance, a deposit of lymph will be observed to form."

But why hypnosis, when a conscious act of attention is "sufficient to change the physical action of the part"?

A Common-Sense View of the Mind Cure 49

Where poison has entered the blood, the out look is not encouraging. Yet Professor Gates has shown by his "Wonder-Bottle" that emotional states change the character of the blood, and it is almost too well known to mention that grief, fear, despondency, and disappointment turn the hair white.

During the siege of Orleans, so the story runs, the soldiers of the Prince of Orange who were afflicted with scurvy were cured by a trick (practically suggestion)—no medicine being available.

It is not generally known that the Yogis of India possess a remarkable control of the body. They have the power to annul pain, and practised feats of levitation, walking on water, etc., centuries before the time of Christ. One of their number who visited Europe and America about five years ago demonstrated to physicians in both countries his ability to stop his heart's action for five seconds at a time—at least so the papers stated.

This, however, has been paralleled in the West. Dr. Brown-Séquard, of Paris, relates that he had a student in one of his classes who could diminish or accelerate his pulse at will. And Dr. Tuckey in "Psycho-Therapeutics" gives, on the authority of Dr. Cheyne, an account of the experiments of a Colonel Townsend. This gentleman, in the presence of physicians, diminished his heart-action until it ceased entirely, and the physicians, after the usual tests, decided that the experiment had been carried too far. But as they were about to leave the room, signs of returning life appeared, and not long after, the heart was beating in a normal manner.

And thus we begin again at the beginning; we do not yet know to what extent the mind may control the body. Because a certain thing has never been done is no reason for assuming that it never will be done. Back to prehistoric cave-dwelling man, rude and unlettered, fashioning his rude implements of clay, is a far cry; and compared with it the civilization of which we boast seems a wondrous thing. Yet it has been compassed solely by the developing brain and mind of man. He has dominated the lower orders of living creatures; he has girdled the earth; who doubts that he will navigate the air? He is harnessing the forces of nature and bending them to his service.

It seems hardly probable that if man can thus control forces external to himself, he is to remain forever subject to forces at work in his own organism. We can not assume that he has reached the climax of his powers—the goal of evolution—and if not, then he will continue to develop mentally.

And this development must certainly give greater self-knowledge and self-command. At the present the average man regards himself as a purely material being—of his mental life and power he has little cognizance. But when he awakes to this self-knowledge, there will follow inevitably an increase of mental power. And thus one may venture to prophesy that through an ever-growing consciousness
of power may man find his way at last to an absolute spiritual dominion, not only over nature but over self.

Mind-cure has been traced to Epidamus, an Egyptian priest, who flourished 500 years before the Christian era. Following him came the Hebrew prophets, who, it is said, also raised from the dead. Then came Jesus and His apostles, whose practises were followed by the priests of the Greek Church until the eleventh century.

In medieval times appeared St. Patrick the

A Common-Sense View of the Mind Cure 51

Apostle, and also the monk Gassner, who healed by touch, as did likewise some of the kings of that age.

In the seventeenth century Valentine Greatrakes, of Ireland, created great excitement; tho hardly greater, perhaps, than did Mesmer, in the last quarter of the eighteenth century, in Paris.

The cures effected by the metallic tractors in England, the "Shriners" of London, "Dr." Cullis of Boston, and the Mormon Elders are comparatively recent; while the miracle, faith, and prayer cures, hypnosis, Christian Science, and New Thought are current history.

A study of these various forms of cure discloses two facts: First, that practically every known disease has been cured by one or another, or so claimed. How permanent such cures were we have no means of knowing. And, second, that all such cures were effected by "a change in the mentality" or a change in the "state of mind." Without this, the cure could not have been wrought.

The only logical conclusion which can be deduced from these facts is that disease is mental or of mental origin.

Every sensible person knows that there is no healing virtue in the bone of some long-defunct saint (even if it can be proved that the bone was once a part of the anatomy of the saint!), but if the sufferer believes that touching it or kissing it will cure his disease, the cure takes place. And if he believes that he is cured, then the disease must have been mental. And if all diseases have been cured by some such means—that is, a change in the mental state—then all disease must be mental.

But, it may be objected, such a disease as consumption can not be mental, because it is induced by bad sanitation.

Let us look at this. St. Paul said, "Man has a natural body and a spiritual body"; but this is equivalent to saying that man is a two-sided phenomenon, both mental and physical. Yet mind and body form a unit, "indissolubly associated," so far as this life is concerned, and because of this unity constantly reacting each part upon the other. So that not only do mental states affect the physical, but the converse; and this unfailing and inevitable interaction brings about, in case of disease, what has been termed "a vicious circle."

Thus, tho a mental state may induce disease, on the other hand the body, reacting upon unhygienic conditions, may also induce disease.

The medical fraternity says that we are constantly taking into the system from the air, water, and food millions of poisonous germs, which, immediately they have gained entrance into the blood, set about to destroy us. But just as a nation maintains a standing army to repel invaders, so nature provides for this contingency by maintaining in the blood millions of other small bodies which attack and destroy the invaders. So long as the vitality or vital force is at par, they do their work well; but if the vital force is lessened by any cause (and bad sanitation among other things will do this), they are no longer equal to the contest and the germs gain the victory. The blood then becomes poisoned, the nutrition of the brain is impaired, and disease follows.

So whether the cause be mental or environmental, the result is the same, as has been said. Therefore diseases which result from unhygienic conditions or the violation of nature's laws can not be said to be mental, or so it seems. But since all disease affects the mental state, it would seem to be closer to the fact to say that all diseases have a mental element.

This is the position taken by a leading London physician and author, and, if true, then all diseases are to some extent amenable to mind-cure. And this would explain why such diseases as consumption have been cured by a "change in the mentality," if it can be shown that such cures were authentic.

It is, however, undeniable that a large number of ills may be traced to mental or nervous origin, and to these one may certainly apply a rational mind-cure, such as has been suggested in these pages.

In chapter first it was pointed out that the organized or classified ideas which constitute the mind are constantly reacting upon the body through the brain and nervous system, thus tending to bring about a mental and physical correspondence. Then if a "change in the mentality" or mental state is all that is necessary to cure disease, the problem is simple enough. One has merely to change his "state of mind," uproot pernicious, and transplant therapeutic, ideas.

But, it may be objected, this is a very slow process; it takes years for the habit of thought to write itself upon the body. This is perfectly true. One may "right about face" in his thinking, strive to ignore pain, divert his mind, and still have ample time to die of the disease before appreciable results are realized. Such a method of self-help presents a fine example of moral courage, will-power, and self-control, all fundamental and necessary; yet in serious or chronic cases it appears to fall short of the mark for these reasons.

In the first place, a persistent effort of will must be made to control the thinking, lift oneself out of the "slough of despond," and ignore pain. It demands unusual self-control, hence such a disciplined mind and will as few persons possess; and, unhappily, pain by its very nature tends to unbalance the mind, thus weakening the power of self-control.

And again, will, like every other mental and moral faculty, has a physical basis. To put it into operation, therefore, requires both moral and what we are accustomed to call physical stamina. But if the brain is in a state of exhaustion, its reaction upon the mind will be feeble, and hence sufficient energy will not be set free to carry out the behest of the mind. It is, of course, possible to whip up the brain by force of will; but it is like whipping up a jaded horse—his little spurt of energy is followed by a still greater exhaustion.

Evidently, then, the slow physical realization of a changed habit of thought and of maintaining the correct mental and moral attitude in really serious disorders gives the problem a disheartening aspect. But when we take into consideration the physical side of the phenomenon called man, we get another point of view. If man were a disembodied spirit, then certainly the cultivation and exercise of his mental and moral faculties should keep him immune to disease. But he has a "natural body," played upon like all the phenomena of nature by natural forces, upon which he reacts; and the manner of this physical reaction is of vital importance. We have already seen that it is effected through the brain and nervous system; but the integrity of the nervous system depends primarily upon the integrity of the brain; hence there must be a normal condition of the brain if we are to obtain the best possible physical reaction.

A carpenter can not build a house with faulty

tools nor a pianist give an artistic performance upon a decrepit piano; and just so the finest, strongest mind can not manifest if its medium, the brain, is debilitated, disorganized, or diseased.

Rational mind-cure, therefore, is of a twofold character: the mental state or mode of thought must be reformed, and the brain must be built up, or brought to the normal standard. Since the fundamental essentials of health are "a sound brain [cortex] and a buoyant mind," we are justified in assuming that those diseases which are not of subjective or mental origin, or due to the entrance of poison into the blood, may be traced to some organic change in the brain structure. For we have it on high authority that "the surest way to check disease is to stimulate the brain [cortex] and increase the mental energy."

The first step in rational mind-cure is unquestionably to change the mode of thought; but it is not enough to stop thinking depressing thoughts—a positive attitude must be taken in order to render the mind buoyant. And this may be done in several ways:

The method of "suggestion "—the daily affirmation of ideal health, hope, and courage—is good, for the reason that the mind feeds upon such ideas as harmonize with the inherent instinct of self-preservation. One is working with nature.

The use of the imagination is equally good; it is a molding force. But it requires mental concentration, which few practise or fully understand, and therefore the simple self-suggestion is easier, generally speaking.

The spiritual uplift which we call prayer is also an aid. For whatever uplifts the soul exhilarates the mind, and we thus get a better mental reaction. Its effect, however, is temporary, and it can not be relied upon to effect a cure; else why were not our martyred presidents restored to health?

Finally, one may try to cultivate a saner philosophy of life. Most of us are too self-centered; we dwell too much upon our personal discomforts. If therefore we can bring ourselves to see that suffering in some form is the common lot; that it is a part of the discipline of life, which chastens the soul and fits it for a nobler sphere of thought and action, we shall go far toward cultivating a cheerful stoicism in regard to our ills.

The second step in self-help is to reform the mode of life, thus securing a better adjustment to external conditions. And here are needed common sense and self-control. The man who persistently fritters away his energy in emotional excesses; who delivers himself up to self-indulgence; who deprives himself of fresh air, sunshine, sleep, pure food, and pure water, or who works each day to the point of exhaustion, must suffer the penalty. The law of compensation can not be escaped. The dyspeptic who persists in "bolting" his food, overloading his stomach, or eating when fatigued can not be cured by any method known to man. If you should have a sore on your hand and removed the scab as fast as it formed, how long would it take for the sore to heal?

Finally, one must by a combined mental and physical treatment build up the brain and thus improve the vitality.

To begin with, the brain is the hardest-worked part of the body, and the tendency of our time is to overwork it. So then one should learn to rest the brain. When the first symptoms of fatigue appear, stop; throw yourself back in an easy chair or couch and relax the muscles. This takes the tension off the brain. Every one knows that when the leg muscles begin to ache, after walking some distance, how refreshed he feels after a halt of a single moment. Having relaxed the muscles, close the eyes, and let the thoughts drift; or, better still, make the mind a blank. Five minutes, even three minutes, will prove refreshing, and it should be resorted to at frequent intervals daily in nervous exhaustion. The celebrated Dr. Pepper, of Philadelphia, trained himself to fall asleep for two or three minutes at frequent intervals throughout the day, and thus accomplished a vast amount of work without fatigue. Just to relax the muscles, hold the brain steady, and stop thinking gives this cerebral rest.

The second measure, both hygienic and mental, is stimulating the brain, but this involves the third, which is breathing.

Some men and nearly all women breathe improperly. With the latter, tight clothing which crowds the vital organs together and diminishes lung space, and the wrong habit of sitting and standing, are responsible. Only a small portion of the lungs is used, and there is residual air which is rarely changed. And yet "breath is life." We can live a number of days without food, several days without water, but only a few moments without air.

Every schoolboy knows that the oxygen in the air is necessary to life. Coming into contact with the blood through the thin membrane which lines the air-cells of the lungs, it changes the impure, blue blood into clean, red blood which pulses through the arteries, carrying the needed elements of nutrition to every part; and it not only cleanses but vitalizes the blood. Therefore, if one desires thoroughly to build himself up, body and brain, he must learn to breathe.

It should be made a habit. If one is obliged to live an indoor life, he should make it a practise to go to the door or window at frequent intervals and take each time at least seven full, deep inhalations, filling the lungs to their utmost capacity. With head erect, and chest lifted, hold the inspired air for a few seconds, to extract all the oxygen from it.

An excellent exercise is to place the feet side by side, clasp the hands, and inhale and exhale regularly for several moments. The brain is thus electrically charged.

Another: Stand erect, inhale deeply, then holding the breath drop the head forward slightly, clench the hands, and tense all the muscles. This stimulates the circulation of the brain.

For nervous debility and mental depression, deep breathing is unexcelled, particularly if one applies imagination. Thus: when inhaling imagine that you are taking into your system the life-giving oxygen; that the invigorated blood is circulating in the brain, stimulating the exhausted cells, and imparting to them new life. With a little practise, one will soon be able to perceive the quickened circulation, which will be followed by a sense of exhilaration.

Local self-treatment comes next in order. We have seen how the vital force leaving the brain spreads throughout the body by means of nerve-fibers; that it is the life-stimulus, since it keeps the internal fires burning; that if it depreciates or is unequally distributed, the weakest spot will be the first to suffer; and that only through its activity can the circulation be kept normal and also the nutrition of each and every part.

Manifestly, then, it is necessary to get control of this life-energy; and it is by no means as difficult as at first appears.

Simply concentrating the attention or fixing the mind upon any organ or part will, as before explained, direct the vital current to that spot. The nerves (vasomotor) will be quickened into action, and the blood-vessels will fill with an excess supply of blood. And as the blood contains the elements of nutrition, an improvement in nutrition will take place. Changes will be made in the chemistry of the secretions, and in the thermic and lymphatic functions. This becomes apparent to the experimenter by the nervous agitation and the sensation of heat. Sometimes there will be a prickling of the skin, or it will "twitch" or "crawl," and again the throbbing of the blood in the arteries may be perceived.

If one applies imagination or "suggestion" results are quicker. Thus: One may form a mental picture of the vital force directed to a given spot, as the gardener turns his hose at will upon the plants under his care, and one may follow in imagination the course of the blood. And, finally, the purpose of all this: a mental picture of the desired result.

It takes longer in the saying than the doing. For once the practise is initiated, the laws of association and habit reinstate previous conditions with astonishing ease. A little practise will bring any part of the body into almost instant communication with the mind.

As the physical processes are automatic it is well to work at regular intervals. Advantage is thus taken of the tendency to reinstate previous experience, and the worker will soon notice the state of preparedness of both mind and body. Ere long the initial impulse will serve to set the train in motion.

It means work—daily, persistent work—to get results. But if pills and powders fail to cure you, what are you going to do about it? Live at a "poor dying rate" or muster up courage to take a hand in your own salvation?

The time required to secure results depends upon the conditions of life, the age, the temperament, and the mental idiosyncrasy of the individual. Obviously success in any field of effort is achieved the more quickly the more enthusiasm and persistence one brings to it.

In most cases, it is wiser to cooperate with a progressive physician—one who is broad-minded enough to recognize the mental factor in disease, and knows how to take advantage of it.

Life is very complex; it is a balancing of many forces and the adjustment of the organism to each and every one. Therefore many things have to be taken into consideration: heredity, temperament, environment, the mental attitude and the constitution, the age, the cause of the existing condition, etc.; and these the physician ponders and weighs as it is possible for very few of the laity to do. One may be working in the dark, when the knowledge of a single fact might put him on the right track.

Again, tho medicine does not always have the expected effect—sometimes a very different one from that anticipated—the patient will find that the effect of such medicine as the modern, up-to-date physician may consider necessary will be greatly intensified by the mental and physical treatment outlined in these pages.

Finally, the action of one mind upon another is more immediately potent than the reaction of the mind upon itself; it is true of all suggestions or impressions received from without. The rose which

I see and smell produces a far stronger effect upon my brain and mind than the rose I imagine I see and smell; that is, an ideal rose.

Thus, you may say to yourself daily: "I am well, and not only am I well, but I feel well. Disease is mental; so if I think myself well, I am well," etc.

Now this undoubtedly tends to buoy up the mind and you feel better in consequence. In course of time, if persisted in, it will bring about an improvement in the physical condition.

But suppose you meet a friend on the street. You are not feeling well, and you know that you look as you feel; nevertheless, when your friend exclaims, with a brightening glance: "How well you look! Why I never saw any one improve as you have! Haven't you gained flesh?"—the effect is magical. You feel instantly better and even doubt that you looked or felt bad in the first instance.

On the contrary, suppose that your friend exclaims with anxiety and dismay written in every line of his countenance: "How bad you look! Aren't you any better? Can't the doctors do anything for you?" Your courage drops below zero at once, and with it goes your vitality; and the idea that you are ill fastens its tentacles upon your mind with an unyielding grip. You not only feel worse, but you are worse. For some one has wisely said: "We think as we feel and we feel as we think we feel."

Hence it is not surprizing when our friends in the kindness of their hearts inquire in doleful accents and grief-drawn faces as to our rheumatism or neuralgia or jaundice that we part company with them in a chastened and despondent frame of mind.

It is, however, a matter which each person must

decide for himself—whether or not he has the necessary knowledge and courage to attack his case single-handed. Some friend or physician may put him on his feet, but, when all is said, the permanence of his cure depends upon himself; for if he drops back into the old habit of thought and life, he will gradually reinstate the conditions which first laid him low, and will naturally relapse into a similar state. He is wise, therefore, in any event, if he sets about his own regeneration.

Moreover, it is a fine discipline for the mind. It strengthens the will, develops self-reliance, self-control, and self-confidence. And when the victory is won, it is virtually self-mastery.

And "whoso conquereth his own soul is greater than he who taketh a city."

A FEW PRACTICAL APPLICATIONS

HEADACHE.—This is usually due to nervous collapse (of the brain), and this causes a derangement of the circulation. The blood congests or stagnates in the membrane which lines the brain.

The obvious treatment is to stimulate the brain and bring the circulation to the normal.

First, open the window, then lie down on the back, with the feet as high as the head and relax the muscles; this takes the tension off the heart and brain.

When the body is completely relaxed, begin to inhale long, deep breaths, regularly, and suggest or imagine that the blood is passing out of the head and to the feet; follow the course of the blood in imagination.

The primary effect is to intensify the pain because more blood rushes to the head; but if the treatment be persisted in for twenty to thirty minutes, the circulation will be regulated; and no congestion, no headache.

There should be continued relaxation and breathing for a half-hour or less, during which one should stop thinking, and let the brain rest.

With intermittent headaches there should be a daily relaxation and treatment until they are brought under control. If there is great debility of the brain and sympathetic centers, this may take several years; it depends upon the age and general condition.

As there is usually more or less derangement of the stomach and liver in such cases, an excellent hygienic measure is to wash out the stomach with hot water on first rising and whenever the stomach is empty.

CONSTIPATION.—This requires local treatment. Concentrate the attention upon the bowels, placing the hands upon them. Hold the mind steady and affirm or imagine that nervous force is passing to the parts; that the increased activity of the nerves will fill the blood-vessels with blood, and that therefore the intestinal muscles will be stimulated to action; that this will free the bowels and keep them free.

At first there will be a sensation of heat, and sometimes pain; but a half-hour treatment, or in some cases less, for a week, will prove efficacious, and if persisted in until tone has been restored to the nerves will forever avert the use of cathartics.

As all the involuntary activity of the body is automatic, regulate movements by the clock. Fix upon a certain hour and expect relief. After one has "got in practise" he will find it possible to stimulate the action of the liver in the same way.

A hygienic measure is copious drafts of water. Children are rarely constipated because of the free use of water. If a pint of water, hot or cold, be drunk on first rising, and a glass or more every time the stomach is empty, the intestinal canal will be "flushed" and the membrane kept clean.

COLDS.—One "takes cold" only when the vitality is low. Anxiety, mental strain, despondency, and fatigue are some of the causes of lowered vitality. A sudden chill contracts the pores of the skin, stops insensible perspiration, and through its action upon

A Common-Sense View of the Mind Cure   65

the sympathetic center deranges the circulation, causing the blood to stagnate in the membrane which lines the air-passages of the head and throat.

It should be arrested in its incipient stage. "An ounce of prevention is worth a pound of cure."

As soon as the symptoms are perceived begin at once to take full, deep breaths, and keep it up. This tends to hold the circulation normal, and no congestion, no cold. Assist the circulation with the imagination and set the will against the cold. An act of will stimulates the brain, and increases the mental energy so that you have more strength to fight the cold.

Open the bowels; if you drink hot water freely, it will tend to do this, and also keep up the temperature.

Eat very little, if at all, until the cold is under control; one needs all his vital force to conquer the cold, and a full stomach needs energy with which to digest the food.

CATARRH.—This is a devitalized condition of the nerves (vasomotor) of the mucous membrane which lines the air-passages of the head and throat, due to numerous past colds. It becomes constitutional because of the passing into the blood of the bacilli in the mucous matter secreted by the membrane. Treatment should be inaugurated by taking a tonic for the blood prescribed by a physician.

The psychophysical treatment is deep breathing of fresh air to build up the brain and improve vitality, and concentration of attention upon the mucous membrane. Stimulating the nerves will improve the circulation and eventually restore tone to the membrane.

If the general condition is much below par, it will

take several years to effect a cure; otherwise, a decided gain will accrue in a few months.

NERVOUSNESS, NERVOUS EXHAUSTION, AND NEURASTHENIA.—These disorders are due to a debilitated brain. The mind should be held calm, and care and worry put aside; above all, fatigue should be avoided. Absolute rest is demanded, mental and physical. Since the brain is the organ of mind, the more one thinks the more one uses the brain; hence one should learn to vegetate "like the cattle on a thousand hills."

Lie out of doors in the sunshine, with muscles relaxed and mind at rest, and breathe, full and deep, hours at a time. Get control of the circulation by imagination and send an excess supply of blood to the brain.

The exercises already described may also be used to advantage.

INDIGESTION.—This is one of our commonest ailments, and those who suffer from it will find by observation that worry, mental strain, despondency, disappointment, and fatigue invariably increase the discomfort. It is oftener the quantity, rather than the quality, of the food which causes distress, and the mode of life is also of moment.

If it is to be overcome, the taint, sometimes hereditary, must be wiped out of the mind and brain. Since it has a depressing effect upon the mind, suggestion and will must be employed to throw off the incubus. Diverting the mind at mealtime and after, cheerful society, laughter, and fresh air, are valuable aids. "Brooding" is especially to be avoided.

Also the brain and sympathetic nerves should be toned up by habitual deep breathing.

For the local treatment: Direct the mind to the

stomach, placing the hands upon it. Take two or three long breaths and at the same time imagine that the vital force is flowing to the part, kindling the nerves to action. Suggest, if you like, that the blood-vessels are filling with blood; that your stomach is strong and fully capable of digesting the food you eat, etc.

If you concentrate your mind well, you will shortly perceive a sensation of heat, and perhaps a quivering of the nerves. After a few moments, the feeling of fulness, weight, and cold will pass off, and very probably gas, if there is fermentation.

This process will have to be repeated daily for an indefinite period to effect a cure, but one can always modify distressing symptoms by such measures.

It goes without saying that if one eats slowly and masticates thoroughly, he will do much toward aiding the other forms of treatment.

RHEUMATISM AND NEURALGIA.—In chronic cases the blood contains an acid for which medical treatment is demanded.

The low nervous state, as in gout, is due to the debility of the brain, sometimes caused by organic changes. Both hygienic and mental treatment should be added to the medical.

Deep breathing, sun-baths, and copious drafts of water are valuable in toning up the brain and nervous system.

As no distinction can be made between a mental and a nervous pain, a strenuous attempt should be made to get control of the mind. Fear of the pain and the "expectant attention" should be overcome. By means of suggestion, daily practised, one may in a few months more or less mitigate the receptivity of the brain (cortex) and the mental sensibility. If one takes hold of it, mentally, when the first symptoms appear, he may by proper suggestions succeed eventually in driving it off. It takes practise, however.

FUNCTIONAL DISORDERS OF WOMEN.—Those incidental to middle life are caused by organic changes taking place in the brain and sex-organism. Nature alone can effect a cure, but the multitudinous discomforts may be mitigated by hygienic and mental treatment.

Recreation will do much toward mitigating mental depression.

Sun-baths, riding and walking, and abundant sleep are hygienic necessities. Water should be drunk freely, to keep the alimentary canal clean and the bowels open.

Deep breathing, more than any other agency, must be relied upon to keep the blood vitalized and the nutrition of the brain normal.

Overwork, mental strain, anxiety, and all depressing emotions should be avoided. A determined effort must be made to be cheerful; tho the sufferer does not feel cheerful, if an attempt is made to appear so, she will tend to become so by a psychological law.

Daily relaxation should be practised—lying on the back, stop thinking, and rest . the brain.

If some new pursuit is taken up, like the study of art or music, botany or floriculture, a new zest is given to life, and the physical ills may be forgotten or relegated to second place.

As the ovaries are leading factors in the disturbances, all other symptoms being mainly reflex, local treatment should be used.

Fix the attention upon the ovaries, placing the hands thereon for a short time daily, and by suggestion and imagination improve the circulation.

A beneficial effect upon the sympathetic centers will thus be produced.

As much as possible the sufferer's mind should be diverted from herself. She should stedfastly refuse to talk about her ailments; and when her attention is called to herself, she will do well to form a mental picture of herself as radiantly well.

FALLING HAIR.—This results from poor circulation in the scalp; insufficient blood-supply deprives the hair-follicles of the elements of nutrition. Daily concentration of attention upon the scalp will put an end to this condition, and new hair may be grown if the hair-glands have not been destroyed by bacilli.

Selected parts of the body may be built up by the psychophysical process so often described.

It can not be dogmatically affirmed that new tissue can be added at will to any part of the body; it is a matter which individual experiment alone can determine. The conditions of life, the mode of life, the age, and assimilative capacity may one or all prevent success.

LEANNESS.—This may be overcome, provided there is no malnutrition or emaciating disease, by holding steadily in "the mind's eye" a picture of what one wishes to become. The experimenter should fix upon the number of pounds to be gained and see the figures as often as possible mentally. If they are written or printed and placed where they may be often seen, it will expedite the result, as will also deep breathing.

SUPERFLUOUS FLESH.—This may be sloughed off in the same manner in which leanness is overcome. In this case, the experimenter should fix upon the number of pounds to be lost. He should live with the mental picture which he creates by suggestion and imagination.

In addition, there should be deep breathing to improve the vitality—excessive flesh denotes an abnormal condition.

In such cases the energy generated by the brain is largely used in converting the food eaten into flesh-forming products. The scholar, the thinker, whose mental life is intensely active, is nearly always of spare figure—the energy is consumed by his mental processes. The restless, nervous person who is constantly turning from one form of activity to another is also thin. The day-laborer, whose mind-action is slight, consumes his energy in muscular exercise. But the good-natured, easy-going individual, who takes life with a cheerful philosophy, and exercises neither his mind nor his muscles to any great extent, is quite sure to take on flesh. The accumulation of fat about the heart, particularly if the vital organs are squeezed together by tight clothing, obstructs the breathing and circulation, hence the blood becomes poor. Many fleshy people have an anemic look.

So, then, the mental energy set free by the brain must be consumed by exercise, mental or muscular, to keep the weight of the body normal.

Women especially need to cultivate deep breathing and take more open-air exercise.

SLIGHT STRUCTURAL DEFECTS.—It is strongly probable that slight structural defects like outstanding ears, round shoulders, or a misshapen nose may be remedied by psychophysical treatment, provided such work is undertaken before the age of thirty. The act of attention improves nutrition, as has been shown, and imagination is a power which we have hardly yet begun to reckon with.

MENTAL STRAIN.—One of the crying evils of

our time is a kind of nervous frenzy—the mad haste to get somewhere or do something; the ambition to get rich, to break records, to win championships, to do the maximum of work in the minimum of time—in short, to compass the impossible.

As a consequence, nervousness, nervous exhaustion, and a long train of ills afflict constantly increasing numbers.

This anxious haste puts a strain upon the mind, which reacts upon the brain and nervous system with deadly effect. Few see it, but nevertheless this mental strain consumes the vitality, exhausts the brain, and if persisted in will finally leave its victim a nervous wreck. Some of the "kings of finance" can not sleep or digest the simplest food.

Many persons attack their daily work under this tension. The thought of the work to be done, the unconscious fear that it may not all be accomplished in the prescribed time, puts the tension on the mind, and this keys up the brain. Ordinary fatigue is thereby increased to exhaustion, and it is an exhaustion of the brain, which frequently induced spells ultimate prostration.

The remedy is simple. One has but to realize the insanity of such a course and calm his mind by an effort of will. A little common-sense mental discipline will break the habit, and the gain in health, self-control, and mental poise will be of lasting value.

"What doth it profit a man if he gain the whole world and lose his own soul?"